WHOLENESS IN CHRIST

WHOLENESS IN CHRIST

DOROTHY VINCENT

CONTENTS

CHAPTER 1

Introduction to Wholeness in Christ

The essence of wholeness in Christ as a spiritual path to health and wellness is the core theme I hope to convey in this essay. In our contemporary era, which professes to value Christian spirituality as a significant asset for health, it is crucial for the followers of Christ to efficiently highlight the importance of hesychasm and Orthodoxy. These elements, like Christianity itself, are not commodities for sale but are profound ways of life aimed at discovering true life. It is essential to note that religions arrived relatively late in human history, and the early Christian Fathers reveal that health and wellness within Christianity are not about mere "feeling good" or materialistic pursuits. As Henri Nouwen critiqued in 1975 regarding the church in the United States, "I had hoped that the vehicle was of the Spirit, but it's really of rationalism and Platonic idealism." Unfortunately, these words still resonate within many of our churches today.

There is a profound interest in Christian spirituality in our contemporary society. However, the writings of mainstream Christian authors on this subject often do not receive the respect or acknowledgment they deserve in the non-Christian world, including both the public sphere and the secular academic realm. Many mainstream Christian writers might share my sentiment that much of our Christian publishing is perceived more as "how-to" manuals focused on personal order and moralism rather than as heart matters deserving deep and authentic reflection. These reflections should encompass all aspects of our lives, including our diverse personalities, varying thoughts, transfigured and disfigured emotions, cognitive and transcognitive actions, as well as moral and ethical values at both soul and depth levels.

Despite the non-Christian world's lack of acknowledgment for contemporary Christian spirituality, my research over the past three years into the contemporary near-death experience (NDE) literature—deliberately excluding NDE accounts by Christian writers—provides compelling evidence. This evidence suggests that NDEs clearly demonstrate experiences of spirit and heart matters that reside in the hearts of all people, irrespective of religion or culture. These experiences often include profound encounters with God's love, universal life reviews, and DMT (the so-called spirit molecule in the brain) experiences.

Defining Wholeness in a Christian Context

Wholeness is a concept defined across various philosophical, religious, and cultural traditions. However, this paper focuses on defining "wholeness" within a Christian context. Within this mainstream denomination, followers are instructed to love and strive to become one with Christ to "be made whole." Thus, our definition of wholeness encompasses spiritual transformation, living in the spirit of Jesus, and becoming more like him to live life as fully and richly as possible. The term "whole" was intentionally chosen over "healed" or "well" because the latter terms often emphasize sickness, unhealthiness, or recovery from trauma.

Wholeness also signifies the interconnectedness of mind, spirit, and body. In the context of early 2020s Christianity, prayer and praying are fundamental practices indicating the habit of relating with God, the Holy Trinity. The spirituality discussed here is a journey toward becoming "more complete" in Christian growth over time, implying that this spirituality is beneficial for overall wellness.

The terms "Christ" and "Jesus" are often used interchangeably in various Christian practices and denominations that pioneer these spiritual pathways to health, healing, and wholeness. While "the God of..." often refers to Christ, "the Spirit of Jesus" is used to refer to the Holy Spirit. This broad usage of terms allows for inclusivity, encompassing followers of New Thought, the "Course in Miracles," unity-affiliated persons, and some non-traditional Christian spiritualists.

CHAPTER 2

Understanding the Connection Between Spirituality

In our quest for greater peace, health, and contentment, many individuals have turned to spiritual practices. There's a growing body of literature emphasizing the powerful alliance between spirituality and health. This paper delves into the insights that historical, philosophical, and theological traditions offer concerning this connection. While we place less emphasis on specific religious beliefs and behaviors, we focus more on the general structures of human well-being and the underlying concerns that drive the pursuit of wholeness. Nonetheless, religious belief forms the core of many spiritualities, highlighting its importance when assessing the various facets of spirituality's impact on health and well-being.

Spirituality, which addresses the ultimate roots of human reality, connects deeply with the concepts of wholeness and health, which in turn address fulfillment in the human condition. Core Western religious texts often link health to a properly ordered existence, an idea accepted by many contemporary health advocates. Historically, human reality was perceived in terms of three intertwined dimensions: body, mind, and spirit. Each dimension required its own development, with a focus on ensuring that body, mind, and spirit were properly coordinated. Despite modern secular voices that continue to address health across all dimensions of human experience, there remains debate on how best to achieve this. The literature on holistic health is extensive, yet there is little consensus on what it means to treat people "holistically." Consequently, the fundamental theological and philosophical reasons for relating wholeness and health have been somewhat overshadowed by debates over the efficacy of specific holistic health models.

Historical Perspectives on Spirituality and Healing
Introduction: Albrecht Dürer's "The Mouth of Truth"

The relationship between spirituality and health in contemporary culture is not a new phenomenon. As we will explore in these pages, similar interests have emerged throughout various historical periods, particularly when health and religious hegemonies began to lose authority. The forces for and against spiritual healing and spiritual paths to health and wellness have waxed and waned in the West since the time of the Greeks.

This chapter provides a historical and contemporary context of the relationships between spirituality and medicine in the United States and Europe. We will also elaborate on the similarities and differences between Eastern and Western spiritual health systems, providing explanatory frameworks for understanding the history, practices, values, and beliefs of various spiritual healing systems.

Throughout history, spirituality has significantly influenced health and healing traditions. In ancient societies, priests and shamans were the primary healers. Over time, Western society developed healthcare traditions among the Greeks, where men of science and the priests of Asclepius became the primary healers. Spirituality was not entirely neglected; in ancient Greek times and the Roman Empire, folk healing practices, particularly through the shrines of Asclepius and the amphitheater at Ephesus, served as both religious and therapeutic centers.

In many healing systems and traditions worldwide, such as those in Africa, Asia, and the Americas, spiritual beliefs and practices have consistently played dominant roles, even before the advent of modern medical science. These traditions underscore the enduring connection between spirituality and health, a connection that continues to be relevant in contemporary discussions on holistic health and wellness.

CHAPTER 3

Biblical Foundations for Health and Wellness

Deuteronomy 30:19-20 (NRSV) speaks of the two paths of life and death, capturing a fundamental biblical theme about God's desire for humanity. Each day, our choices form us into the image of God or in our own image. Jesus, seen as a profoundly healthy person and miracle worker, emphasized teaching, preaching, and healing both sin and sickness. God transformed the apostle Paul, making him whole and well, prompting Paul to advocate for the holistic salvation offered by God in Christ Jesus. This positions physical and spiritual well-being as natural partners in God's plan for wholeness. Various biblical foundations support the concepts of health and wellness.

According to Vine's Expository Dictionary, "Health" is defined as "the state of being sound and whole; properly to be fit," whereas "Wellness" is defined as "the quality or state of being in good health, especially as an actively sought goal." Paul, in his letters, elaborates that Christian communities are a temple. Theologian Sallie McFague interprets this not as a prohibition on substances like alcohol and drugs, which did not exist in Paul's era, but as an exhortation advocating self-care. Paul understood that many in the 1st century

Ephesian congregation would have been alcohol users, making it implausible for him to simply forbid drinking altogether. Instead, he likely encouraged drinking in a controlled and responsible manner. Given the anatomical and psychiatric vulnerabilities of former alcoholics, it is commonly recommended to err on the side of caution. This nuanced understanding pertains to consuming wine during the 1st century when the risks were not fully comprehended.

Key Scriptures on Wholeness and Well-Being

Numerous scriptures speak to the fundamentals of holism, emphasizing the importance of body, mind, and spirit as equally vital dimensions of our humanity. These scriptures provide a solid foundation for understanding the spiritual paths to health and wellness outlined in the New Testament. There is a profound belief in Jewish and Christian scriptures that one's relationship with God is deeply connected to one's relationships within our human networks. The Torah, or law in Judaism, sets precedents to promote ethical and holy relationships among the Children of Israel and Yahweh. This divine guidance extends to aspects of health.

Ironically, modern times have seen some elements once dismissed as woo-woo, like biblical salt, found to have medical validity. While we may not view scriptures purely as preventative medicine, their advice should be considered divinely inspired and therefore holy. The Old Testament teaches the desolation brought by sin and disease (e.g., Deuteronomy 28; Leviticus 26). The consequences of sin under the Covenant are either death and doom or, as Isaiah 38 puts it, a call to repent to avoid losing one's blessings. In both scenarios, health is intrinsically linked to our relationship with the Eternal.

In the Apostolic church, health was not a primary issue; however, healing patterns were established through acts at the Council of Jerusalem and leadership letters to the churches. These guidelines remain valid for the church today, continuing to underscore the connection between spiritual practices and health.

CHAPTER 4

Prayer and Meditation as Spiritual Practices for H

There is a growing body of evidence suggesting that spiritual beliefs and practices are closely linked to better health and personal wellness. Prayer and meditation, integral components of these practices, are often cited as powerful tools for maintaining health and well-being. When individuals engage in frequent prayer or maintain a personal spiritual or religious connection, they often report reduced stress levels, fewer visits to physicians, and quicker recovery times from illness. In a Christian context, prayer often involves reading scripture, either privately or with others, and using physical symbols of faith. Private prayer, in particular, involves interior communication and serves as a search for support and a continual awareness of one's relationship with God, fostering a partnership with the divine.

Effectiveness of Prayer and Meditation in Holistic Health

The effectiveness of prayer and meditation as part of a holistic health regimen is multifaceted. Studies often focus on individuals facing prolonged health challenges rather than life-threatening diseases. It is crucial to recognize that spiritual health often serves as a vital area of strength for these individuals. Belief in God can provide a strong foundation for healing across a range of neurological, behavioral, biological, financial, and peripheral challenges. The faith, trust, hope, and meaning that come from a spiritual partnership provide relief and equilibrium in the face of pain and adversity. While perception can influence the experience of pain and reduce the body's overall physiological response, pain still serves a survival function by compelling behavior modifications to avoid harm.

The Power of Prayer in Healing

Few aspects of the spiritual journey toward wellness generate as much controversy as praying for health. For some, prayer is seen as a superstitious relic that has no place in modern medicine. For others, it is viewed as a mental crutch effective through the placebo effect. Years ago, I attended a United Methodist Episcopal Conference focused on the Book of James and the healing ministry of Jesus within the church. At one point during the conference, a woman in a wheelchair was brought out, and we were asked to pray for her as a demonstration of our belief in healing prayer. Despite her condition remaining unchanged during the meeting, the pervasive atmosphere of spiritual excitement and healing vitality left a lasting impression.

Research into the power of prayer for healing often highlights the elusive nature of its efficacy. As Robert Eliot notes in his comprehensive work, *The Power of Prayer on Getting Well*, it is challenging to "prove" prayer's effectiveness in a research setting. The act of prayer involves an intuitive approach, relying on the faith of those praying rather than measurable outcomes. Despite sixty years of research by scholars like Elizabeth Targ, George Gallup, and Larry Dossey, the precise mechanism by which prayer contributes to healing remains unclear. Statistical experiments cannot reliably predict specific outcomes from focused prayer. So why study it? As Eliot argues, "because we want to know how to alleviate suffering." For those dismissing placebo studies as merely legal narcotic peddling or negative spiritualism, the research on prayer, albeit controversial, remains a valuable and ongoing field of inquiry.

CHAPTER 5

Embracing Mind-Body-Spirit Integration

As human beings, we are a trinity of mind, body, and spirit. We are composed of both material and non-material elements. Our experiences and functions are rooted in our physical bodies, yet they transcend into the realm of the soul. Modern medicine increasingly acknowledges the importance of healing our bodies in connection with healing our souls. Simultaneously, we discover that by caring for our bodies as children of God, our hearts and spirits can also heal. Unfortunately, many wellness routines focus strictly on the surface level, which often leads to their failure.

The Importance of Holistic Self-Care in Christian Spirituality

Considering holistic self-care is crucial for Christian spirituality, integrating care for the mind, body, and spirit. The positive practical values of learning your body habits and healing routines are numerous. Such knowledge empowers you to maintain a balanced lifestyle that enhances overall well-being. Furthermore, embracing a holistic approach to self-care aligns with Christian teachings of nurturing the body as a temple of the Holy Spirit.

A personal spiritual belief or experience that beckons one toward caring for mind, body, and spirit together might include the understanding that achieving harmony in all aspects of life reflects the divine order and leads to a more fulfilled existence. For example, prayer and meditation can strengthen your spiritual connection, promote mental clarity, and offer emotional balance, which in turn supports physical health.

Holistic Approaches to Well-Being

As mentioned in earlier sections, the integration of body, mind, and spirit continues to gain momentum across religion, psychology, and medicine. Holistic (or whole-person) approaches to wellness encompass various practices that contribute to overall well-being. Practices linked directly to medicine, such as mindful breathing exercises, and those connected to spirituality, like cultivating a sense of the sacred or seeking union with a higher power, both aim to integrate the self, fostering a sense of wholeness.

Christian wellness and spirituality are often promoted through multiple channels: personal and professional literature, community and support groups, local and international congregations, nondenominational fellowship groups, and medical and psychological clinics and programs. This widespread promotion underscores the importance of addressing the interconnected dimensions of health.

An individual's spirituality should align with their ultimate beliefs, values, and priorities. Christianity, often interpreted as a spiritual path toward greater self-discovery and self-actualization, also serves as an expression of adoration, faith, and dependence on a higher power. Changes in therapeutic practices and evolving societal understandings of wellness and health have led medical personnel and mental health care providers to give increased attention to patient spirituality. In 2008, for example, the Joint Commission declared that a patient's spiritual needs are just as important and should be assessed and treated as seriously as their physical and mental/emotional ailments.

Holistic approaches to wellness and health aim to provide a comprehensive understanding of personhood. Worldview training, such as that offered by Christianity, serves as an intervention to help practitioners enable individuals to thrive. Embracing a holistic perspective ensures that we address the entirety of the human experience, fostering a balanced and fulfilling life.

Community and Fellowship in Promoting Health

Support systems and community play a crucial role in making us whole and healthy. Research over the past thirty years has consistently shown that social support is a key variable influencing various health states. People are inherently aware of the need for connection and community. For instance, thirty years ago, most married men who had heart attacks experienced them at home, often in bed on a Sunday morning, highlighting the connection between heart attacks and stress. As smoking has decreased and been identified as a major factor in heart disease, the incidence of heart attacks in middle-aged men has shifted. Today, those who suffer from heart attacks often do so from Monday to Friday between 8-9 A.M. Studies with men who have had heart attacks reveal that chronic social stress at home and work is a significant predictor of heart disease and diabetes, underscoring the link between stress and illness.

The Role of Faith and Fellowship in Reducing Stress

Total wellness, or health, is a central theme of this discussion. Too often, we view health and wellness promotion at an individual level. As Christians, we are not isolated entities; we are interconnected and create community. Much of the New Testament emphasizes wholeness, teaching that reconnection with God and neighbor leads to wellness. Paul provided healthy guidelines for living, including: don't criticize, don't tear others down, don't look for faults or failings, assume the best, and maintain a positive attitude.

To promote wellness, churches should include small group ministries, self-help groups (for diabetes, smoking cessation, battered women), and mutual therapy groups within their circles of concern. Churches and their leaders often do not view their ministry as therapeutic, but an expanded view that includes education can enhance this perception. For our purposes, we will use the terms mutual therapy and support groups interchangeably. Reducing stress involves avoiding isolation and focusing on community wellness. By reintroducing wellness services, Christian ministers can significantly enhance the health of their congregations.

The Role of Church and Community Support

One of the intangible but powerful animators of wellness is the sense of belonging that comes from being part of a community. Connection with the church and community can lead to cellular-level changes, including immunological fluctuations. Pastors now encourage parishioners to attend worship services and participate in church school classes, support groups, educational programs, Bible studies, and social activities. The practical and spiritual reasons for this encouragement include the numerous benefits of faith community support: it significantly contributes to health and wholeness, listening helps us grow, being prayed for transcends scientific measurement, and serving strengthens both ourselves and others.

The story of free health screening and nutrition information provided to community clients illustrates the characteristic of wellness promotion. Those living in the Anamchara community recall their wholeness as they connect with the reign of God—a reign sometimes difficult to express in words but tangible in the healer's role in life. This is evident in the nurse's office filled with pictures of the community, Chapel of St. Brigid nurse's logos, and symbols of wholeness like the circle. All these elements convey a profound message of belonging, free of forced relationships or guilt.

CHAPTER 7

Overcoming Barriers to Wholeness

Attempts to integrate spiritual aspects into mental health counseling, diet and weight control, chemical dependency counseling, and other wellness programs have faced various barriers. These barriers exist at individual, professional, political, and institutional levels. Many health professionals are hesitant to include spiritual orientations in their work due to the diverse, ambiguous, and often unclear definitions of spirituality, leading to numerous symbols and stigmas. This fear persists despite the potential benefits of integrating spirituality into health practices.

Barriers to Integrating Spirituality in Healthcare

Religious beliefs or traditional practices connected to spirituality in healthcare typically involve some form of divine or external services. Professionals often question people's past experiences, social values, capacity for interaction, knowledge of medicine, and understanding of the holistic dual functions of the human body. Health or mental health practitioners may lack the skills to know where to start or how to access religious counseling and offer depth. This fear often stems from ignorance, and raising awareness requires a combination of diagnostic and commercial strategies. Practitioners must consider the clinical process and ethical implications to effectively use spiritual routes in health, necessitating a thorough exploration of spirituality.

Addressing Stigma and Misconceptions

Stigma and misconceptions can prevent individuals from accessing the mental health care they need, especially when linked to stereotypes of violence associated with mental illness. Indeed, 51% of British Columbia residents report feeling uncomfortable talking with people who have a mental illness; 14% would try to avoid them.

Historically, the Church has often presented individuals with mental illness as "possessed by the devil" or morally deficient. Over time, most churches and their members have learned that mental illness is a health issue that should be treated as such. However, increased knowledge and understanding of mental illness have not eliminated the social stigma it carries. Many factors contribute to the negative stereotypes, misconceptions, and avoidance behaviors toward individuals with mental illness, with media portrayal being one of the most influential.

The Role of Media in Shaping Perceptions

Media is a critical tool for publicizing important health issues and can significantly influence how people think and feel about mental illness. Misconceptions about mental illness are prevalent among the general public, including followers of Christ. This is why confidential resources that are not associated with formal mainstream organized religion but operate from a Christ-centered point of view are so important. These resources can provide a supportive environment for individuals seeking mental health care without the fear of judgment or stigma.

Practical Steps for Integrating Spirituality in Health Care

To integrate spiritual aspects into health care effectively, practitioners need to take several practical steps:

1. **Education and Training**: Health professionals should receive education and training on the importance of spirituality in health and wellness. This training can help them understand how to incorporate spiritual practices into their care plans and address the unique needs of their patients.
2. **Collaborative Approach**: Practitioners should adopt a collaborative approach, working with religious leaders and spiritual counselors to provide comprehensive care that addresses the physical, mental, and spiritual aspects of health.
3. **Creating Supportive Environments**: Health care facilities should create supportive environments that encourage the exploration of spirituality. This includes providing spaces for prayer and meditation and offering resources that support spiritual growth.
4. **Awareness Campaigns**: Public awareness campaigns can help reduce stigma and misconceptions about mental illness and the role of spirituality in health. These campaigns should highlight the benefits of integrating spiritual practices into health care and provide information on available resources.
5. **Confidential Resources**: Establishing confidential resources that offer spiritual support from a Christ-centered perspective can help individuals feel more comfortable seeking care without fear of judgment.

Conclusion

Overcoming the barriers to integrating spirituality into health care requires a concerted effort from health professionals, religious leaders, and the broader community. By addressing stigma and misconceptions, providing education and training, and creating supportive environments, we can promote a holistic approach to health and wellness that recognizes the importance of mind, body, and spirit.

CHAPTER 8

Caring for the Whole Person: Practical Application

Introduction

In **Wholeness in Christ: Spiritual Paths to Health and Wellness**, the Health Message Committee of the Wesleyan Church clearly identifies the call to return to our roots in God when treating those who seek our care. We have discovered that there are practical approaches to increasing spiritual depth. Although we may never have all the answers, it is still worthwhile to work toward moving our people toward wholeness.

In our pursuit of wholeness, we recognize the need to develop an interdisciplinary position emerging from existing research on both faith and health. Since physical health contributes to spiritual depth and peace, and spiritual depth correlates with better physical health indicators and mental health, we aim to provide practical avenues for functioning in the present world that care for the whole person.

God is at work in this world, and as co-laborers with God, we partner to work in accord with the style of Jesus. Our immediate challenge is to present theoretical support for the practical concepts mentioned in **Wholeness in Christ**. We will use the following secondary questions to substantiate the podcasts already provided in an earlier clarification essay:

1. What is going on in this world?
2. What is the developing position regarding management?
3. What are the concrete methods to be discussed?
4. Has anyone had any success with the research on faith and health?

In this chapter, we seek an interdisciplinary position on faith and health research, providing not only theoretical support for a practical religious approach but also estimates of its proposed effectiveness.

Integrating Faith and Health in Daily Life

Although living a whole life in Christ may seem elusive in secular medical contexts, individuals can integrate faith and health within Christian settings. A research participant's admonition to "find wholeness in Christ, even when we cannot find a medical cure" suggests that integrating faith and health can be a practical solution for locating spiritual paths to health and wellness.

For example, Natalie, a 34-year-old mother of two, strikes a balance between medico-scientific and faith-based paradigms as she chronicles her difficult pregnancy, which required bed rest and involved heart problems. Natalie shares her experience:

"When I found out about my heart, I was very, very scared of raising these kids... I started stressing out so much that I began to fear what would happen when I gave birth or if I would even make it to the end of the pregnancy. I started falling sick a lot with asthma. We were very active in church, but I stopped attending and began staying home, following God. I started drawing back to Christ. Although I was a Christian, I wasn't dedicated – I had a turning point and made a change in my life. Things just fell into place, I got closer to God, work improved, and I didn't stress as much."

Natalie draws upon faith in the act of surrendering to God and following Him in her daily life as a practice. This way of living keeps intact a whole vision of health and wellness that transcends the materialistic parameters of biomedicine alone. She embodies her faith in the practice of not just being "active" in church but also praying alone, reading the Bible, and making her spiritual devotion palpable in her mothering of pre-born triplets. Natalie's way of being captures the essence of moving from the inside out as a spiritual practice expressed beyond the biomedical paradigm.

"I wasn't taking my medications properly. I was taking them a bit, I wasn't checking my blood, I wasn't watching my diabetes, I was just fading out of what I should be doing."

CHAPTER 9

Conclusion: Embracing Wholeness in Christ

Wellness is a central concern for many people. It is crucial to recognize that treating health and illness in compartmentalized, reductionistic ways leads to misunderstandings. This essay explores wellness through the holistic lens of Christian faith, revealing that true wellness requires a relational approach based on faith, hope, and love. Such a way of life is exemplified in the teachings of Jesus Christ and is nurtured and empowered by the Spirit of the Risen Christ, uniting us with God our Creator and the created world. Both Christ and St. Paul exemplify the principle that body and spirit are unified in practice.

In this essay, we showcased four understandings of embracing wholeness in Christ, as enunciated by Larchet, Ware, and Matthew the Poor. The unchanging use of the Christian sacraments, moral living, service, and life of prayer are four spiritual paths that guide us toward healing and wholeness, which entail authentic wellness. Our task in this life is to focus on and practice all four of these throughout our physical and spiritual existence.

Today's society often overemphasizes the significance of the body and resorts to various forms of compartmentalization. In contrast,

Christians understand that the body is more than just skin and bones; both body and soul require care and nurturing through spiritual ascesis, such as prayer. This worldview allows Christians to perceive health and wellness as holistic blessings emanating from the threefold sharing of the grace of Christ. Wholeness in Christ does not begin with an earthly sacrament; rather, the growth that has begun must continue until the end. All four actions—use of sacraments, moral living, service, and life of prayer—are intertwined and assist in stabilizing our efforts for the better. This holistic approach ensures that we may reach the everlasting life promised at the final severance on the fixed date of our natural death.

Reflecting on Holistic Wellness

Wholeness in Christ is about more than just physical health; it is about integrating all aspects of our being—mind, body, and spirit—into a cohesive whole. This integration allows us to live a life that reflects the fullness of God's creation and the teachings of Christ. By embracing a holistic approach to wellness, we can experience the true depth of health and spiritual well-being.

The Role of Community and Fellowship

Community and fellowship play a vital role in promoting holistic wellness. Being part of a faith community provides the support, encouragement, and accountability needed to pursue a balanced and healthy life. Engaging in communal worship, participating in small groups, and serving others are all ways to foster a sense of belonging and connection, which are essential for holistic health.

Practical Steps for Embracing Wholeness

To embrace wholeness in Christ, we should:

1. **Engage in Regular Prayer and Meditation**: These spiritual practices help us connect with God and nurture our spiritual health.

2. **Participate in the Sacraments**: Regular participation in the sacraments strengthens our faith and fosters a sense of spiritual well-being.
3. **Live a Moral and Ethical Life**: Following the teachings of Christ and living a life of integrity promotes overall wellness.
4. **Serve Others**: Serving others not only benefits those we help but also enhances our own sense of purpose and fulfillment.
5. **Foster Community and Fellowship**: Being part of a faith community provides the support and encouragement needed to pursue holistic wellness.

By integrating these practices into our daily lives, we can move toward a state of holistic wellness that embraces the fullness of God's creation. This approach allows us to experience the true depth of health and spiritual well-being, ultimately leading us to the everlasting life promised in Christ.